Vascular Compression Syndromes - What You Need to Know

Dr. Mohammad E. Barbati

PART ONE
INTRODUCTION

VASCULAR COMPRESSION SYNDROMES

Vascular compression syndromes refer to a group of conditions that occur when a blood vessel is compressed or restricted by an adjacent structure, leading to a variety of symptoms. These syndromes are generally associated with the compression of nerves or vessels, and they can be caused by a variety of anatomical and physiological factors.

To understand vascular compression syndromes, it is important to first understand the anatomy and physiology of the affected structures. Blood vessels are responsible for transporting blood throughout the body, while nerves are responsible for transmitting signals between the brain and various parts of the body. In some cases, blood vessels and nerves run near each other, and this can lead to the compression of one or both structures.

There are a variety of vascular compression syndromes that can occur, depending on the location and extent of the compression. Some of the most common types of vascular compression syndromes include thoracic outlet syndrome

(TOS), popliteal artery entrapment syndrome, nutcracker syndrome (NS), median arcuate ligament syndrome (MALS) and May-Thurner Syndrome (MTS).

The symptoms of vascular compression syndromes can vary depending on the specific condition, but they typically involve pain, weakness, and/or numbness in the affected area. Diagnosis of these syndromes can be challenging, as the symptoms can be vague and nonspecific. However, a thorough medical history and physical examination, along with imaging studies such as ultrasound or magnetic resonance angiography (MRA), can help to make an accurate diagnosis.

It is important to note that the symptoms of vascular compression syndromes can mimic those of other conditions, such as carpal tunnel syndrome or peripheral artery disease. Therefore, it is important to consider a wide range of differential diagnoses when evaluating patients with suspected vascular compression syndromes.

THE CONTROVERSY OF VASCULAR COMPRESSION SYNDROMES

Even though vascular compression syndromes have been recognized and studied for many years, there is still some controversy surrounding their existence. Some experts argue that these syndromes are over diagnosed and that many patients are undergoing unnecessary and potentially harmful treatments. Others contend that these syndromes are under diagnosed and that many patients are suffering needlessly due to a lack of awareness and understanding.

One of the main arguments against the existence of vascular compression syndromes is that they are often diagnosed based on imaging studies alone, without considering the patient's clinical symptoms. Some experts believe that the presence of vascular compression on imaging studies does not necessarily mean that the patient is experiencing symptoms, and that these findings may be incidental and not clinically significant.

Another argument against vascular compression syndromes is that they are often treated with invasive procedures, such as stent implantation or angioplasty, that carry their own risks and complications. Some experts argue that these treatments should only be used in cases where the patient is experiencing significant symptoms and that more conservative approaches, such as physical therapy or pain management, should be tried first.

On the other hand, supporters of vascular compression syndromes argue that they are often under diagnosed and that many patients are suffering needlessly due to a lack of awareness and understanding. They point out that the symptoms of these syndromes can be vague and nonspecific, and that they may be misdiagnosed as other conditions.

Proponents also argue that the diagnosis of vascular compression syndromes should be based on a combination of imaging studies and the patient's clinical symptoms. They contend that imaging studies can provide valuable information about the location and extent of vascular compression, but that the patient's symptoms are ultimately the most important factor in determining whether treatment is necessary.

Finally, proponents argue that the risks and complications of invasive treatments such as stent implantation or angioplasty are often outweighed by the potential benefits in patients who are experiencing significant symptoms. They point out that these treatments can be highly effective in alleviating symptoms and improving quality of life, and that they should be considered as a viable option for patients who are not responding to more conservative treatments.

The controversy surrounding the existence of vascular compression syndromes continues to be a topic of debate among medical professionals. While some argue that these syndromes are over diagnosed and that many patients are undergoing unnecessary treatments, others contend that they are under diagnosed and that many patients are suffering needlessly. Ultimately, the diagnosis and treatment of vascular compression syndromes should be based on a careful evaluation of the patient's clinical symptoms and imaging studies, with the goal of providing the most effective and appropriate care possible.

PURPOSE OF THE BOOK

The purpose of this book is to provide a comprehensive overview of vascular compression syndromes, including their causes, symptoms, diagnosis, and treatment. Through a detailed examination of the latest research and clinical practice guidelines, this book aims to provide non-healthcare professionals with the information and tools they need to know about these conditions.

PART TWO
ANATOMY AND PHYSIOLOGY

OVERVIEW OF VASCULAR ANATOMY AND PHYSIOLOGY

Understanding the anatomy and physiology of the vascular system is essential for diagnosing and treating vascular compression syndromes. This chapter provides an overview of the vascular anatomy and physiology, focusing on the structures and processes relevant to vascular compression syndromes.

The vascular system consists of a network of blood vessels that transport oxygen and nutrients to the body's tissues and organs. It is divided into two main parts: the arterial system and the venous system.

The arterial system carries oxygenated blood away from the heart and delivers it to the body's tissues and organs. Arteries are thick-walled, muscular vessels that have a pulsatile flow due to the pressure generated by the heart. The largest artery in the body is the aorta, which branches into smaller arteries that supply blood to specific regions of the body.

The venous system carries deoxygenated blood back to the

heart. Veins are thinner-walled and less muscular than arteries, and they have a slower, non-pulsatile flow. The largest vein in the body is the inferior vena cava, which receives blood from the lower half of the body and delivers it to the right atrium of the heart.

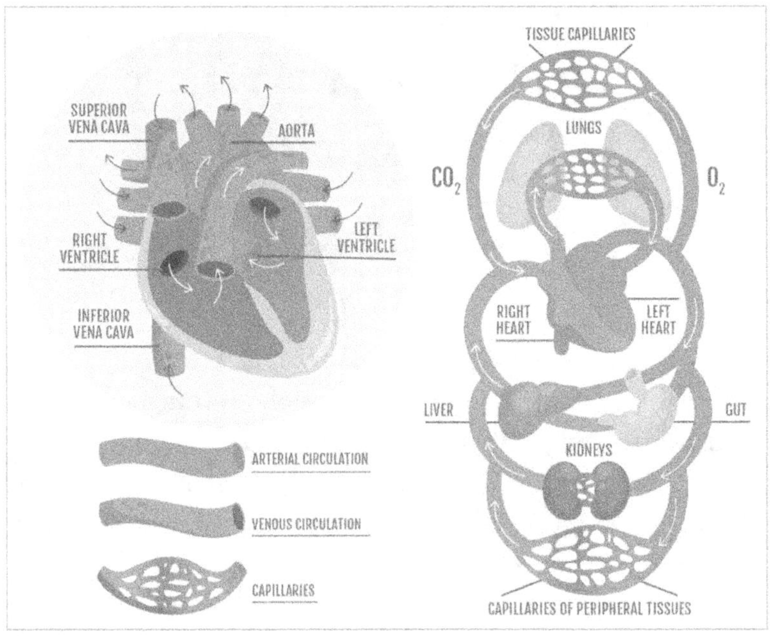

Vascular compression syndromes can occur when blood vessels are compressed or narrowed by surrounding structures, such as bones, muscles, or other blood vessels. This can lead to a reduction in blood flow, which can cause a range of symptoms depending on the location and severity of the compression.

The diagnosis and treatment of vascular compression syndromes require a thorough understanding of the anatomy and physiology of the vascular system. Imaging studies such as ultrasound, magnetic resonance angiography (MRA), and computed tomography (CT) scans can provide detailed information about the structure and function of the blood vessels, which can help guide treatment decisions.

THE ROLE OF NERVES AND VESSELS IN VASCULAR COMPRESSION SYNDROMES

Vascular compression syndromes are often caused by the compression or entrapment of blood vessels or nerves by surrounding structures. Understanding the role of nerves and vessels in these syndromes is crucial for accurate diagnosis and effective treatment.

Nerves play a vital role in the regulation of blood vessel tone and blood flow. When nerves are compressed or entrapped, they can disrupt this delicate balance, leading to changes in blood flow and tissue perfusion. In addition, nerve compression can cause a range of symptoms, including pain, numbness, and weakness.

One example of a vascular compression syndrome caused by nerve entrapment is thoracic outlet syndrome (TOS) . This syndrome occurs when the nerves and blood vessels that supply the arm are compressed as they pass through the thoracic outlet, a narrow passageway between the neck and the chest. Symptoms of TOS can include pain, numbness, and weakness in the arm and hand, as well as headaches and neck pain.

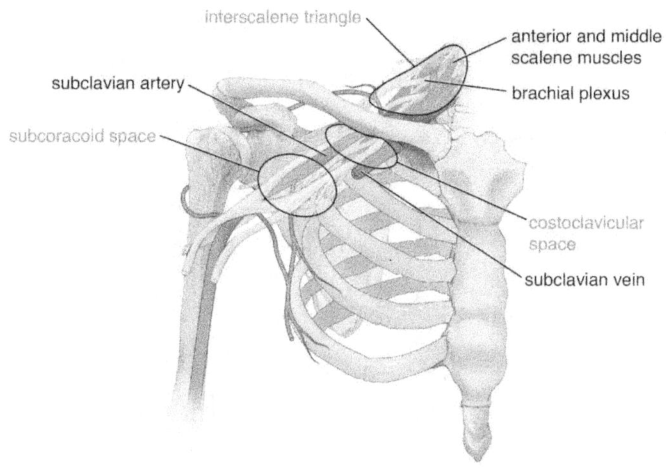

Another example of a vascular compression syndrome caused by nerve compression is median arcuate ligament syndrome (MALS). This syndrome occurs when the median arcuate ligament, a band of tissue that connects the diaphragm to the spine, compresses the celiac artery and the nerves that supply the stomach and intestines. Symptoms can include abdominal pain, nausea, and vomiting.

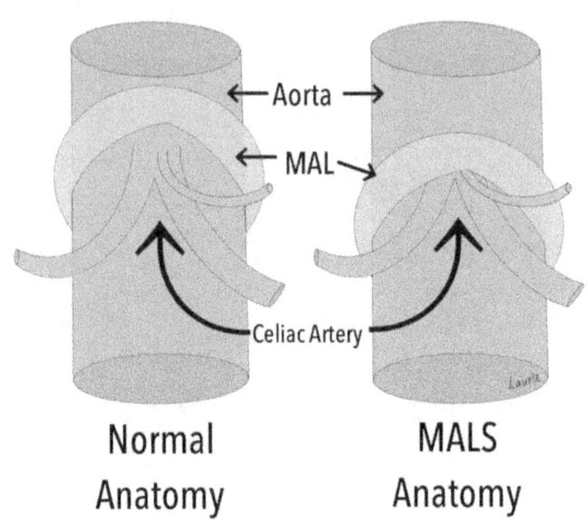

Another example of a vascular compression syndrome caused by blood vessel compression is popliteal artery entrapment syndrome. This syndrome occurs when the popliteal artery, which supplies blood to the lower leg and foot, is compressed by surrounding muscles and tendons. Symptoms can include pain, numbness, and weakness in the leg and foot, as well as coldness and discoloration of the skin.

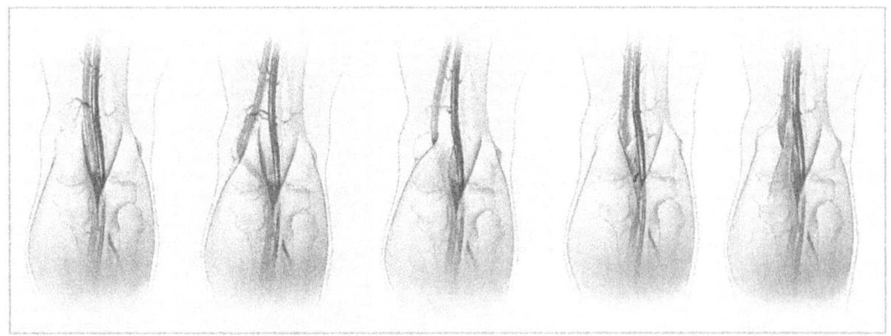

May-Thurner syndrome (MTS) is another example of a vascular compression syndrome caused by blood vessel compression. This syndrome occurs when the left iliac vein is compressed by the right iliac artery, leading to reduced blood flow and the formation of blood clots. Symptoms can include pain and swelling in the legs, as well as an increased risk of deep vein thrombosis.

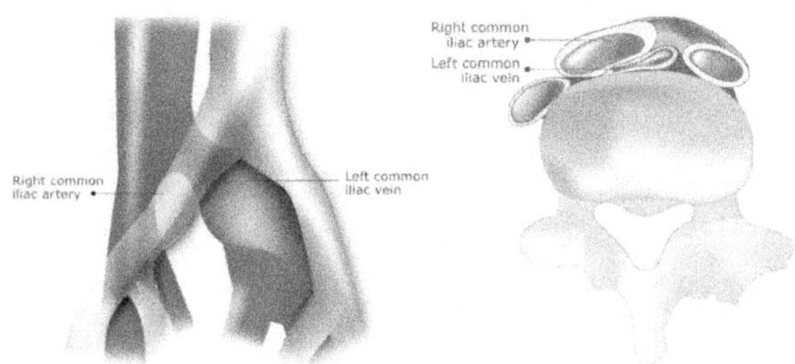

In summary, the role of nerves and vessels is critical in the development of vascular compression syndromes. By understanding the mechanisms involved, healthcare professionals can accurately diagnose and effectively treat these conditions, improving patient outcomes and quality of life.

PART THREE
HISTORICAL OVERVIEW OF VASCULAR COMPRESSION SYNDROMES

EARLY DESCRIPTIONS OF VASCULAR COMPRESSION SYNDROMES

Vascular compression syndromes have been recognized and studied for centuries, with early descriptions dating back to ancient medical texts. In this chapter, we will explore some of the earliest descriptions of vascular compression syndromes and how they have evolved over time.

One of the earliest descriptions of a vascular compression syndrome comes from the ancient Egyptian medical text, the Ebers Papyrus, which dates back to 1550 BCE. The text describes a condition known as "wry-neck," which is now believed to be a form of thoracic outlet syndrome. The Ebers Papyrus describes symptoms such as neck pain, shoulder pain, and weakness in the arm, which are all characteristic of thoracic outlet syndrome.

Similarly, the ancient Indian medical text, the Charaka Samhita, describes a condition known as "Kata Shirsha" which is now believed to be a form of brachial plexus compression. The text describes symptoms such as pain, numbness, and weakness in the arm and hand, which are all characteristic of brachial plexus compression.

In the 18th and 19th centuries, there were several notable descriptions of vascular compression syndromes. In 1768, the Scottish anatomist Alexander Monro described a condition known as "cervical rib," which is now known as thoracic outlet syndrome with a cervical rib.

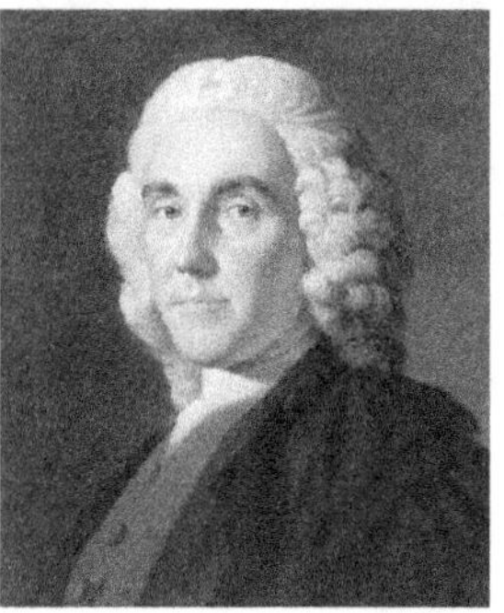

In 1854, the French surgeon Jean-Louis Petit described a condition known as "coarctation of the aorta," which is now believed to be a form of median arcuate ligament syndrome.

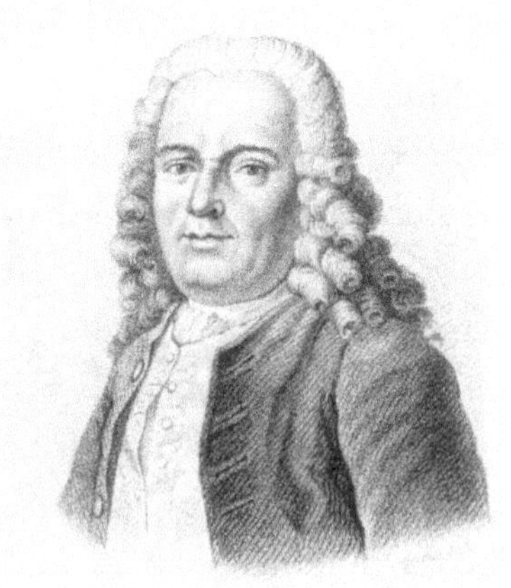

In the 20th century, there was an increasing recognition of vascular compression syndromes, particularly with the development of diagnostic imaging techniques such as angiography and MRI. In 1956, the American surgeon William J. Adson published a seminal paper on thoracic outlet syndrome, in which he described the clinical features of the condition and proposed surgical treatments.

Today, vascular compression syndromes are well-recognized and studied, with numerous publications and medical textbooks dedicated to the subject. However, there is still controversy surrounding the existence and diagnosis of some of these syndromes, as well as the most effective treatments.

EVOLUTION OF THE CONCEPT OF VASCULAR COMPRESSION SYNDROMES

The concept of vascular compression syndromes has evolved significantly over time, from early descriptions in ancient medical texts to our current understanding of the pathophysiology and treatment of these conditions.

As discussed in the previous chapter, early medical texts described symptoms and conditions that are now recognized as vascular compression syndromes. However, these early conceptualizations did not include a clear understanding of the underlying anatomy and physiology of these conditions.

In the late 19th and early 20th centuries, there was a growing understanding of the anatomy and physiology of the cardiovascular and nervous systems. This led to a more detailed understanding of the underlying causes of vascular compression syndromes.

For example, in the case of thoracic outlet syndrome, it was recognized that compression of the brachial plexus and subclavian artery could be caused by a cervical rib or other bony abnormalities. Similarly, in the case of median arcuate ligament syndrome, it was recognized that compression of the celiac artery could be caused by the median arcuate ligament of the diaphragm.

The concept of vascular compression syndromes has evolved significantly over time, from early descriptions in ancient medical texts to our current understanding of the pathophysiology and treatment of these conditions. Advances in medical knowledge and technology have led to improved diagnostic and treatment options, but controversies and challenges remain. Further research is needed to fully understand and address these challenges.

CONTROVERSIES SURROUNDING THE VASCULAR COMPRESSION SYNDROMES

Vascular compression syndromes are complex conditions that can be challenging to diagnose and treat. Despite advances in medical knowledge and technology, controversies and challenges remain surrounding the diagnosis and treatment of these conditions.

CONTROVERSIES SURROUNDING DIAGNOSIS

One of the main controversies surrounding the diagnosis of vascular compression syndromes is the lack of consensus on diagnostic criteria for some of these conditions. For example, the diagnosis of nutcracker syndrome, which is characterized by compression of the left renal vein between the superior mesenteric artery and the aorta, can be challenging due to a lack of clear diagnostic criteria. Some studies have suggested that nutcracker syndrome is overdiagnosed, while others argue that it is underdiagnosed and that there is a need for more accurate diagnostic criteria.

Another controversy surrounding the diagnosis of vascular

compression syndromes is the use of imaging techniques. While angiography and MRA can be useful for diagnosing these conditions, there is debate over which imaging modality is most appropriate and whether imaging should be used as a screening tool or reserved for patients with specific symptoms.

CONTROVERSIES SURROUNDING TREATMENT

Treatment options for vascular compression syndromes can also be controversial, as there is a lack of consensus on which interventions are most effective. In some cases, surgery may be recommended to relieve compression of the affected vessel or nerve, while in other cases, conservative measures such as physical therapy or medication may be sufficient.

One of the main controversies surrounding the treatment of vascular compression syndromes is the effectiveness of surgical interventions. While some studies have reported high success rates for surgical interventions such as first rib resection and scalenectomy for thoracic outlet syndrome, others have reported lower success rates and a high rate of complications. Similarly, the effectiveness of stent implantation or angioplasty for conditions such as May-Thurner syndrome is still debated, with some studies reporting high success rates while others report lower success rates and a high rate of complications.

PART FOUR
CLINICAL PRESENTATION AND DIAGNOSIS

CLINICAL PRESENTATION

Vascular compression syndromes can present with a wide range of symptoms, depending on the location and severity of the compression. Symptoms can be chronic or intermittent and can range from mild to severe. A thorough history and physical examination, along with appropriate imaging studies, can help diagnose these conditions and guide appropriate treatment.

THORACIC OUTLET SYNDROME (TOS)

Thoracic outlet syndrome (TOS) is a condition that results from compression of the brachial plexus and/or subclavian vessels as they exit the thoracic outlet. Symptoms can include:

- Pain in the neck, shoulder, arm, or hand
- Weakness or numbness in the arm or hand
- Swelling or discoloration of the arm
- Coldness or tingling in the arm or hand
- Muscle wasting in the hand

Symptoms of TOS can be aggravated by certain activities, such as reaching overhead or carrying heavy objects.

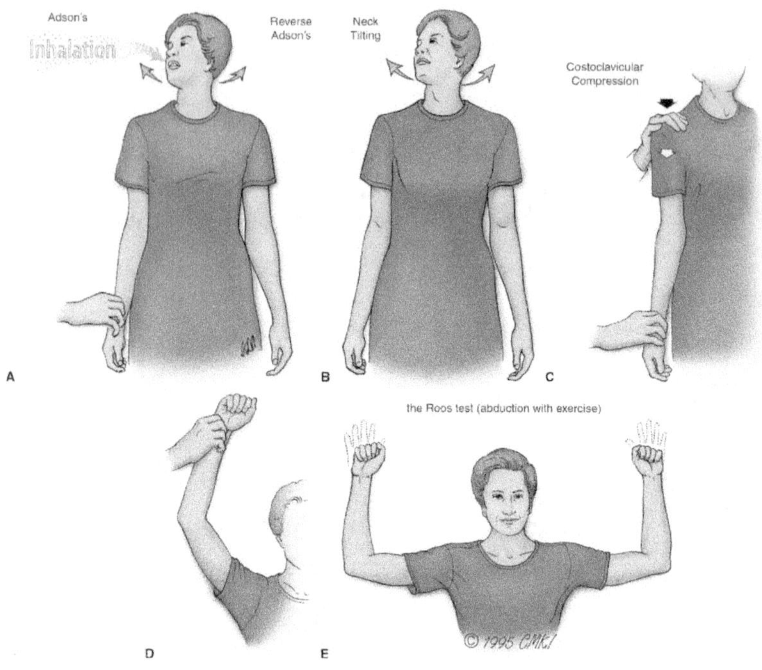

NUTCRACKER SYNDROME

Nutcracker syndrome is a condition that results from compression of the left renal vein between the superior mesenteric artery and the aorta. Symptoms can include:

- Hematuria (blood in the urine)
- Flank pain
- Varicocele (enlargement of the veins in the scrotum)

MAY-THURNER SYNDROME (MTS)

MTS is a condition that results from compression of the left iliac vein by the right iliac artery. Symptoms can include:

- Swelling or pain in the left leg
- Varicose veins in the left leg
- Skin discoloration or ulceration in the left leg

MEDIAN ARCUATE LIGAMENT SYNDROME (MALS)

MALS is a condition that results from compression of the celiac artery by the median arcuate ligament. Symptoms can include:

- Abdominal pain after eating
- Weight loss
- Nausea or vomiting
- Diarrhea or constipation

OTHER VASCULAR COMPRESSION SYNDROMES

Other vascular compression syndromes can present with a wide range of symptoms, depending on the location and severity of the compression. For example, compression of the ilioinguinal nerve can result in pain or numbness in the groin or inner thigh, while compression of the popliteal artery can result in pain or cramping in the calf muscle.

DIAGNOSTIC METHODS

T he diagnosis of vascular compression syndromes can be challenging, as the symptoms can be nonspecific and can mimic other conditions. It is essential to work with a healthcare provider experienced in diagnosing and treating vascular compression syndromes.

A thorough physical examination is the first step in diagnosing vascular compression syndromes. The physician will look for signs of swelling, discoloration, and venous distension in the affected area. They will also check for decreased or absent pulses and evaluate for any signs of neurological deficit, such as muscle weakness or numbness.

Imaging studies are essential in diagnosing vascular compression syndromes. The following tests are commonly used:

ULTRASOUND

Ultrasound is a non-invasive imaging technique that uses high-frequency sound waves to create images of the blood vessels. Ultrasound can detect the presence of venous or arterial stenosis, thrombosis, or compression.

MAGNETIC RESONANCE ANGIOGRAPHY (MRA)

MRA uses a strong magnetic field and radio waves to create detailed images of the body. MRA can be useful in identifying the location and severity of vascular compression, as well as any associated nerve or tissue damage.

COMPUTED TOMOGRAPHY (CT) ANGIOGRAPHY

CT angiography is a non-invasive imaging technique that uses X-rays to create detailed images of the blood vessels. CT angiography can identify the location and severity of vascular compression and any associated complications, such as thrombosis or aneurysm.

ANGIOGRAPHY

Angiography is an invasive imaging technique that involves the injection of contrast dye into the blood vessels. This allows for detailed images of the blood vessels to be obtained, which can identify the location and severity of vascular compression.

NERVE CONDUCTION STUDIES (NCS) AND ELECTROMYOGRAPHY (EMG)

NCS and electromyography EMG are tests that evaluate the electrical activity of nerves and muscles. These tests can be useful in identifying nerve damage and evaluating the severity of nerve compression.

DIFFERENTIAL DIAGNOSIS OF VASCULAR COMPRESSION SYNDROMES

Vascular compression syndromes can present with a wide range of symptoms that may mimic other medical conditions. Therefore, it is crucial to rule out other potential causes before making a definitive diagnosis. In this chapter, we will explore the differential diagnosis of vascular compression syndromes.

DEEP VEIN THROMBOSIS (DVT)

Deep vein thrombosis (DVT) occurs when a blood clot forms in a deep vein, most commonly in the legs. DVT can cause swelling, pain, and redness in the affected area, which may be similar to the symptoms of vascular compression syndromes. However, in DVT, the swelling typically starts in the calf and progresses up the leg, whereas in vascular compression syndromes, the swelling is usually localized.

PERIPHERAL ARTERY DISEASE (PAD)

Peripheral artery disease (PAD) occurs when there is a buildup of plaque in the arteries that supply blood to the legs. PAD can cause pain, cramping, and numbness in the legs, which may be similar to the symptoms of vascular compression syndromes. However, in PAD, the symptoms typically occur during exercise and improve with rest, whereas in vascular compression syndromes, the symptoms may occur at rest and worsen with exercise.

LUMBAR DISC HERNIATION

Lumbar disc herniation occurs when the soft inner portion of a spinal disc protrudes through the outer ring and presses on the nerves. This can cause pain, numbness, and weakness in the legs, which may be similar to the symptoms of vascular compression syndromes. However, in lumbar disc herniation, the pain is usually located in the lower back and buttocks, whereas in vascular compression syndromes, the pain is usually located in the affected limb.

PERIPHERAL NEUROPATHY

Peripheral neuropathy is a condition that results in damage to the peripheral nerves, which can cause pain, numbness, and weakness in the affected area. This may be similar to the symptoms of vascular compression syndromes. However, in peripheral neuropathy, the symptoms may be bilateral and symmetric, whereas in vascular compression syndromes, the symptoms are usually localized to one limb.

The differential diagnosis of vascular compression syndromes includes a wide range of medical conditions that may present with similar symptoms. Therefore, it is essential to rule out other potential causes before making a definitive diagnosis. A thorough medical history, physical examination, and appropriate imaging studies can help differentiate between these conditions and guide appropriate treatment. It is essential to work with a healthcare provider experienced in diagnosing and treating vascular compression syndromes.

PART FIVE
TREATMENT OF VASCULAR COMPRESSION SYNDROMES

CONSERVATIVE MANAGEMENT

Conservative management of vascular compression syndromes involves non-invasive treatments that aim to relieve symptoms and improve overall quality of life. Compression therapy, physical therapy, lifestyle changes, and pain management are all non-invasive treatment options that can be used alone or in combination. It is essential to work with a healthcare provider experienced in diagnosing and treating vascular compression syndromes to determine the best course of treatment. In some cases, conservative management may not be sufficient, and more invasive treatments may be necessary.

COMPRESSION THERAPY

Compression therapy is a commonly used non-invasive treatment for vascular compression syndromes. This involves wearing compression stockings that provide pressure to the affected limb, helping to improve blood flow and reduce swelling. Compression therapy is often recommended as a first-line treatment for mild to moderate cases of vascular compression syndromes.

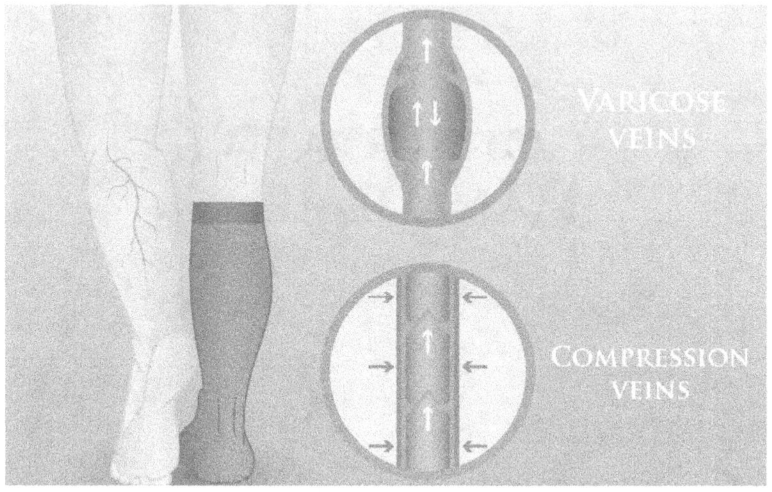

PHYSICAL THERAPY

Physical therapy can help alleviate the symptoms of vascular compression syndromes by strengthening the muscles in the affected area, improving flexibility, and promoting blood flow. Physical therapy may involve exercises to strengthen the muscles, massage therapy, and other manual therapies.

LIFESTYLE CHANGES

Lifestyle changes can also play a role in the conservative management of vascular compression syndromes. Patients may be advised to maintain a healthy weight, quit smoking, and engage in regular exercise to improve blood flow and reduce symptoms. Additionally, patients may be advised to avoid sitting or standing for long periods and to take breaks to move around and stretch.

PAIN MANAGEMENT

Pain management can also be an essential aspect of conservative management for vascular compression syndromes. Over-the-counter pain medications, such as ibuprofen or acetaminophen, can be used to relieve mild to moderate pain. In some cases, prescription pain medications or nerve blocks may be required to manage severe pain.

SURGICAL INTERVENTIONS

Surgical interventions for vascular compression syndromes may be necessary when conservative management is not effective, or symptoms are severe. Venous stenting, lumbar sympathectomy, and first rib resection are all surgical procedures that may be used to treat vascular compression syndromes. It is essential to work with a healthcare provider experienced in diagnosing and treating vascular compression syndromes to determine the best course of treatment. In some cases, a combination of surgical and non-surgical treatments may be necessary to achieve optimal outcomes.

VENOUS STENTING

Venous stenting is a minimally invasive procedure that involves the placement of a stent in the affected vein to improve blood flow. This procedure is commonly used to treat May-Thurner Syndrome and iliofemoral deep vein thrombosis. During the procedure, a thin catheter is threaded through the vein and a stent is placed to hold the vein open. This procedure can be done under local anesthesia and is typically done as an outpatient procedure.

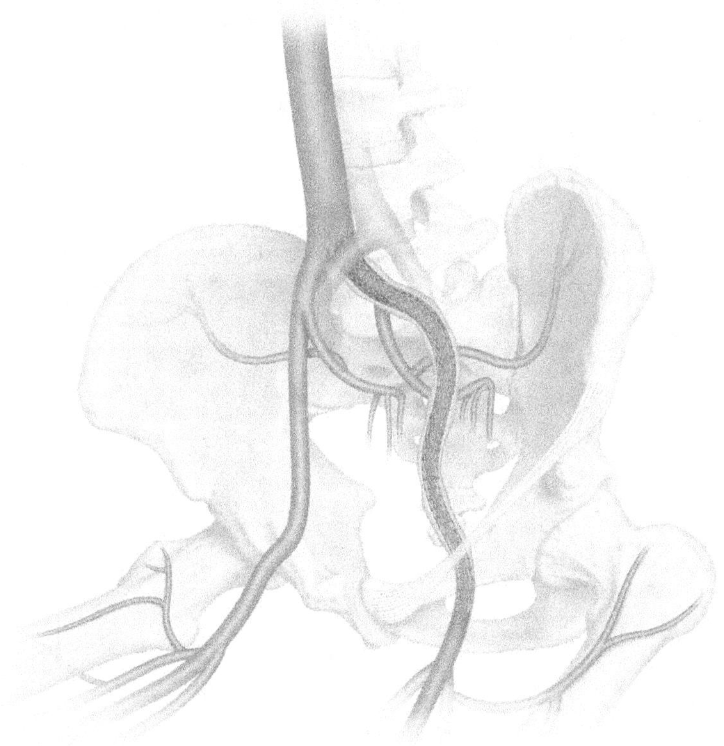

LUMBAR SYMPATHECTOMY

Lumbar sympathectomy is a surgical procedure that involves cutting or clamping the sympathetic nerves that run alongside the spine. This procedure is used to treat conditions such as thoracic outlet syndrome and Raynaud's disease. By cutting or clamping the nerves, blood vessels in the affected area can dilate and improve blood flow. This procedure is typically done under general anesthesia and may require a short hospital stay.

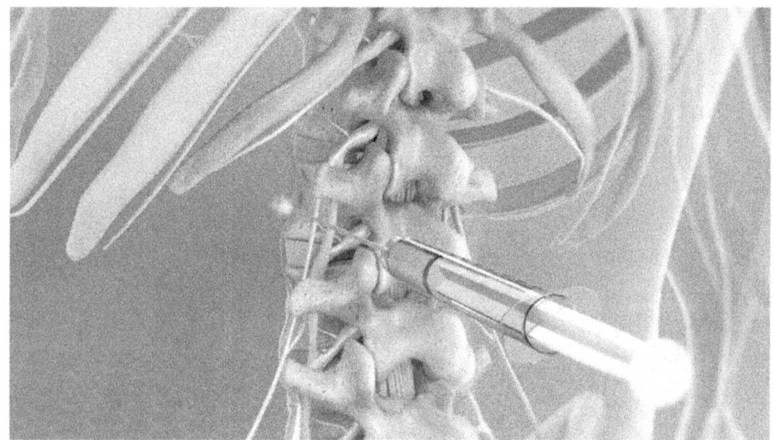

FIRST RIB RESECTION

First rib resection is a surgical procedure that involves the removal of the first rib to relieve compression on nerves and blood vessels in the area. This procedure is commonly used to treat thoracic outlet syndrome. During the procedure, a small incision is made, and the first rib is removed. This procedure can be done under general anesthesia and may require a short hospital stay.

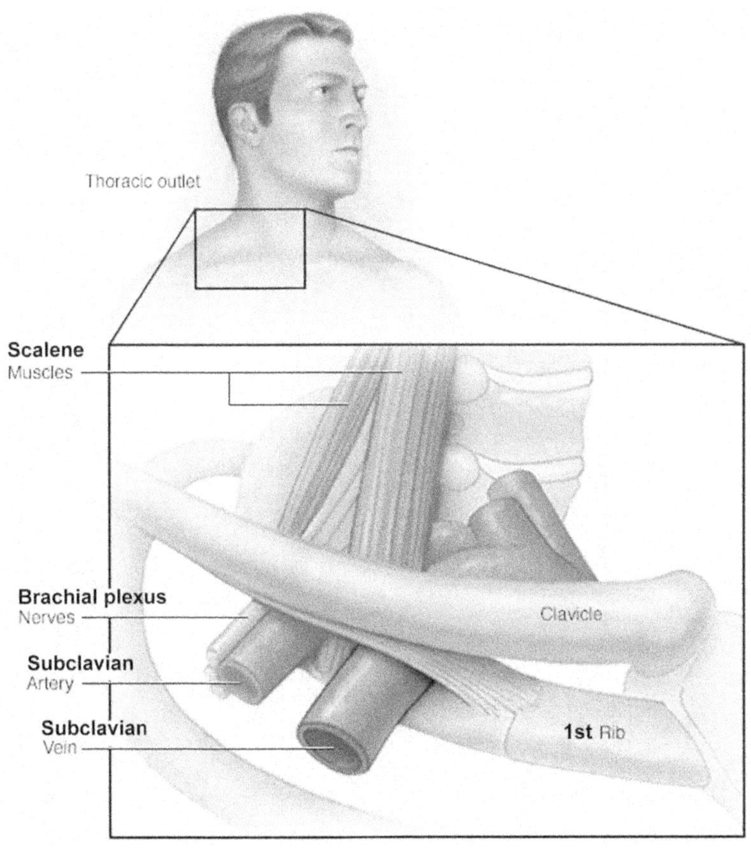

PART SIX
EVIDENCE-BASED RESEARCH ON VASCULAR COMPRESSION SYNDROMES

OVERVIEW OF RESEARCH STUDIES ON VASCULAR COMPRESSION SYNDROMES

In this chapter, we will provide an overview of the current research studies on vascular compression syndromes. Research studies are important to further our understanding of the pathophysiology, diagnosis, and treatment of these conditions.

PATHOPHYSIOLOGY STUDIES

Research studies have explored the underlying pathophysiology of vascular compression syndromes. For example, studies have investigated the role of anatomical variations, such as the presence of a cervical rib, in the development of thoracic outlet syndrome. Other studies have explored the biomechanics of vascular compression and the resulting hemodynamic changes that occur.

DIAGNOSTIC STUDIES

Studies have also investigated the accuracy and reliability of diagnostic tests for vascular compression syndromes. For example, research has evaluated the sensitivity and specificity of imaging tests such as magnetic resonance angiography (MRA) and computed tomography (CT) scans for diagnosing May-Thurner Syndrome.

TREATMENT STUDIES

Research studies have also explored the efficacy of different treatment options for vascular compression syndromes. For example, studies have evaluated the outcomes of surgical interventions such as decompression and revascularization procedures. Other studies have investigated the use of endovascular procedures such as angioplasty and stenting in the treatment of these conditions.

LIMITATIONS OF RESEARCH STUDIES

Despite the important contributions of research studies to our understanding of vascular compression syndromes, there are also limitations to consider. Some studies may have small sample sizes, making it difficult to generalize results to larger populations. Additionally, there may be variations in the diagnostic criteria and treatment protocols used across studies.

CRITIQUE OF THE QUALITY OF RESEARCH STUDIES ON VASCULAR COMPRESSION SYNDROMES

While research studies on vascular compression syndromes have provided important insights into the pathophysiology, diagnosis, and treatment of these conditions, there are limitations and critiques that must be considered. The limited research evidence, variations in diagnostic criteria and treatment protocols, and the risk of bias in studies all pose challenges to the interpretation and generalization of study results. Moving forward, it is important for future studies to address these limitations and conduct high-quality research to advance our understanding and treatment of vascular compression syndromes.

LIMITED RESEARCH EVIDENCE

Despite the prevalence and potential severity of vascular compression syndromes, there is still a limited amount of high-quality research on these conditions. Many of the studies that have been conducted have had small sample sizes, making it difficult to generalize results to larger populations. Additionally, there is a lack of randomized controlled trials (RCTs) investigating the efficacy of different treatment options for these conditions.

VARIATIONS IN DIAGNOSTIC CRITERIA

The diagnosis of vascular compression syndromes can be challenging due to the variability in symptoms and lack of specific diagnostic criteria. This has resulted in variations in the diagnostic criteria used across studies. For example, studies investigating thoracic outlet syndrome may use different diagnostic criteria, such as symptom-based criteria or anatomical criteria, which can lead to inconsistencies in study results.

VARIATIONS IN TREATMENT PROTOCOLS

Similar to diagnostic criteria, there are variations in treatment protocols used for vascular compression syndromes. This can make it difficult to compare the outcomes of different treatment options across studies. For example, studies investigating the efficacy of surgical interventions for May-Thurner Syndrome may use different techniques or variations in the procedure, leading to variations in outcomes.

BIAS

There is a risk of bias in research studies on vascular compression syndromes, particularly in studies evaluating treatment efficacy. This is because many of the studies are observational and not randomized, making it difficult to control for confounding variables. Additionally, there may be conflicts of interest, such as researchers having financial ties to the companies that produce the devices used in endovascular procedures.

FUTURE DIRECTIONS FOR RESEARCH ON VASCULAR COMPRESSION SYNDROMES

Research on vascular compression syndromes is still in its early stages, and there are several areas where future research could provide valuable insights. Large-scale studies, standardized diagnostic criteria, multidisciplinary approaches, long-term outcomes, comparative studies, and patient-reported outcomes are all potential areas for future research on these conditions. By addressing these areas, we can improve our understanding and treatment of vascular compression syndromes and improve patient outcomes.

LARGE-SCALE STUDIES

As previously mentioned, many of the studies on vascular compression syndromes have had small sample sizes, which limits the generalizability of the results. Future research could focus on conducting larger scale studies with larger sample sizes to provide more robust evidence on the epidemiology, diagnosis, and treatment of vascular compression syndromes.

STANDARDIZED DIAGNOSTIC CRITERIA

There is a need for standardized diagnostic criteria for vascular compression syndromes to reduce the variability in the diagnosis across studies. This would enable researchers to compare outcomes across different studies and ensure consistency in the diagnosis and classification of these conditions.

MULTI-DISCIPLINARY APPROACHES

Vascular compression syndromes can involve multiple systems, including vascular, neurological, and musculoskeletal systems. Future research could focus on adopting a multi-disciplinary approach, involving collaboration between vascular surgeons, neurologists, radiologists, and physical therapists, to provide a comprehensive evaluation of these conditions.

LONG-TERM OUTCOMES

Many of the studies on vascular compression syndromes have focused on short-term outcomes. Future research could focus on long-term outcomes, including recurrence rates, quality of life measures, and long-term complications.

COMPARATIVE STUDIES

Comparative studies of different treatment modalities for vascular compression syndromes could provide valuable information on the efficacy and safety of different interventions. This would enable clinicians to make evidence-based decisions on the most appropriate treatment for their patients.

PATIENT REPORTED OUTCOMES

Patient-reported outcomes are becoming increasingly important in healthcare research. Future studies could include
patient-reported outcomes to provide insights into the impact
of vascular compression syndromes on patients' daily lives and
to evaluate the effectiveness of different interventions from the
patient's perspective.

PART SEVEN

CASE STUDIES

The following case studies illustrate the varied clinical presentations, diagnostic approaches, and management strategies for vascular compression syndromes. May-Thurner syndrome, thoracic outlet syndrome, nutcracker syndrome, and popliteal artery entrapment syndrome are just a few examples of these conditions. Early recognition and appropriate management are essential to prevent complications and improve patient outcomes.

CASE 1: MAY-THURNER SYNDROME

A 45-year-old woman presented with a 6-month history of left lower limb swelling and pain. She had no significant medical history and was not taking any medications. Physical examination revealed left lower limb edema, erythema, and tenderness. Duplex ultrasound showed evidence of deep vein thrombosis (DVT) in the left femoral vein. CT angiography revealed narrowing of the left common iliac vein due to compression by the overlying right common iliac artery, consistent with May-Thurner syndrome. The patient was started on anticoagulation therapy and underwent angioplasty with stent placement in the left common iliac vein, which resulted in complete resolution of symptoms and restoration of normal venous flow.

CASE 2: THORACIC OUTLET SYNDROME

A 32-year-old man presented with a 3-month history of right upper limb pain, numbness, and weakness. He had no significant medical history and was not taking any medications. Physical examination revealed reduced sensation and weakness in the right upper limb, with positive Tinel's sign over the brachial plexus. Electromyography (EMG) showed evidence of denervation in the right upper limb, consistent with a neurogenic lesion. MRI of the cervical spine showed no abnormalities. CT angiography revealed compression of the right subclavian artery and vein at the thoracic outlet, consistent with thoracic outlet syndrome. The patient underwent surgical decompression of the thoracic outlet, which resulted in complete resolution of symptoms.

CASE 3: NUTCRACKER SYNDROME

A 28-year-old woman presented with a 1-year history of intermittent left flank pain and hematuria. She had no significant medical history and was not taking any medications. Physical examination was unremarkable. CT angiography revealed compression of the left renal vein between the aorta and superior mesenteric artery, consistent with nutcracker syndrome. The patient underwent laparoscopic left renal vein transposition, which resulted in complete resolution of symptoms.

CASE 4: POPLITEAL ARTERY ENTRAPMENT SYNDROME

A 27-year-old man presented with a 2-year history of right calf pain and cramping during exercise. He had no significant medical history and was not taking any medications. Physical examination revealed a reduced dorsalis pedis pulse in the right foot. Doppler ultrasound showed evidence of popliteal artery stenosis, which was confirmed on CT angiography. The patient underwent surgical release of the popliteal artery, which resulted in complete resolution of symptoms.

PART EIGHT
DISCUSSION OF TREATMENT OUTCOMES AND FOLLOW-UP

The treatment of vascular compression syndromes is complex and requires a multidisciplinary approach. The treatment options for these conditions depend on the severity of the symptoms, the underlying anatomical abnormalities, and the patient's overall health status. In this chapter, we will discuss the various treatment options available for vascular compression syndromes and the outcomes of these treatments.

CONSERVATIVE TREATMENT OPTIONS

Conservative treatment options for vascular compression syndromes include lifestyle modifications, physical therapy, and medications. Lifestyle modifications such as weight loss, regular exercise, and avoiding prolonged periods of standing or sitting can help alleviate symptoms in some cases. Physical therapy can be useful in treating musculoskeletal causes of compression, such as tight muscles or scar tissue. Medications such as pain relievers, anticoagulants, and muscle relaxants can also be used to manage symptoms.

SURGICAL TREATMENT OPTIONS

Surgical treatment options for vascular compression syndromes include decompression surgery, which involves releasing the compressed vessel, and venous reconstruction, which involves repairing or replacing damaged veins. These procedures may be performed through traditional open surgery or minimally invasive techniques such as endovascular surgery. The choice of procedure depends on the location and severity of the compression and the patient's overall health status.

OUTCOMES OF TREATMENT

The outcomes of treatment for vascular compression syndromes can vary depending on the type and severity of the condition, as well as the chosen treatment option. In general, conservative treatments such as lifestyle modifications and medications may provide temporary relief of symptoms but do not cure the underlying condition. Surgery can provide more lasting relief but carries the risk of complications and may not be appropriate for all patients.

For patients who undergo surgical treatment, the success of the procedure depends on factors such as the location and severity of the compression, the surgeon's expertise, and the patient's overall health. Complications can include bleeding, infection, nerve damage, and blood clots. Venous reconstruction procedures may have a higher risk of complications compared to decompression surgery.

Follow-up after treatment is important to monitor for recurrence of symptoms or complications. Patients who undergo surgical treatment should be closely monitored for a period of time after the procedure to ensure that the surgical site is healing properly and that symptoms are improving.

70

PART NINE
LAST WORDS

Vascular compression syndromes are a group of conditions that can cause a range of symptoms and complications. Despite the controversy surrounding their existence, there is a growing body of evidence to support the diagnosis and treatment of these conditions. The purpose of this book was to provide an overview of vascular compression syndromes, including their anatomy and physiology, clinical presentation, diagnostic methods, and treatment options.

Throughout this book, we discussed the various types of vascular compression syndromes, their early descriptions, and the evolution of the concept over time. We also explored the controversies surrounding their diagnosis and treatment, as well as the quality of research studies on these conditions.

While there is still much to learn about vascular compression syndromes, the available evidence suggests that these conditions can be diagnosed and treated effectively. Conservative treatment options such as lifestyle modifications and medications can provide temporary relief of symptoms, while surgical options such as decompression surgery and venous reconstruction can provide more lasting relief.

However, the success of treatment depends on many factors, including the severity of the condition, the underlying anatomical abnormalities, and the patient's overall health status. In addition, the choice of treatment should be made on an individual basis, taking into account the risks and benefits of each option.

PART TEN
RECOMMENDATIONS FOR FUTURE RESEARCH AND CLINICAL PRACTICE

The study of vascular compression syndromes is an evolving field, with new research and developments emerging all the time. In this chapter, we will provide some recommendations for future research and clinical practice in the area of vascular compression syndromes.

Increase awareness and education: One of the main challenges in diagnosing and treating vascular compression syndromes is that many healthcare professionals are not aware of these conditions. More education and awareness campaigns are needed to improve recognition and diagnosis of these conditions.

Improve diagnostic methods: Current diagnostic methods for vascular compression syndromes, such as imaging studies, have limitations and are not always reliable. There is a need for the development of new and more accurate diagnostic methods that can provide clinicians with more detailed information about the anatomy and physiology of the vessels and nerves involved in these conditions.

Develop standardized treatment protocols: There is a lack of standardized treatment protocols for vascular compression syndromes, which can lead to variability in treatment outcomes and patient care. The development of standardized treatment protocols, based on the latest research and clinical evidence, could help improve the quality of care for patients with these conditions.

Conduct more high-quality research: There is a need for more high-quality research studies on vascular compression syndromes, including randomized controlled trials and systematic reviews. Such studies can provide clinicians with more reliable and comprehensive information about the diagnosis and treatment of these conditions.

Collaborate across specialties: Vascular compression syndromes require a multidisciplinary approach, involving specialists from multiple fields, including vascular surgery, neurology, radiology, and physical therapy. Collaborative efforts across these specialties could lead to improved diagnosis and treatment of these conditions.

Develop patient-centered outcomes: Patient-centered outcomes, such as quality of life and functional status, should be prioritized in research studies on vascular compression syndromes. Such outcomes can provide valuable information about the impact of these conditions on patients' lives and the effectiveness of different treatment options.

In conclusion, the study of vascular compression syndromes is a complex and evolving field. Improving diagnosis, developing standardized treatment protocols, and conducting high-quality research are essential for improving the quality of care for patients with these conditions. Collaboration across specialties and prioritizing patient-centered outcomes are also important for improving the overall management of vascular compression syndromes.

ABOUT THE AUTHOR

Dr. Mohammad E. Barbati is a consultant vascular and endovascular surgeon. He obtained an MD in endovascular treatment of venous diseases from University Hospital, Aachen. In 2018 he was appointed as a consultant vascular surgeon and lecturer at University Hospital Aachen. Dr. Barbati has been a principal or co-investigator in several clinical trials and studies involving 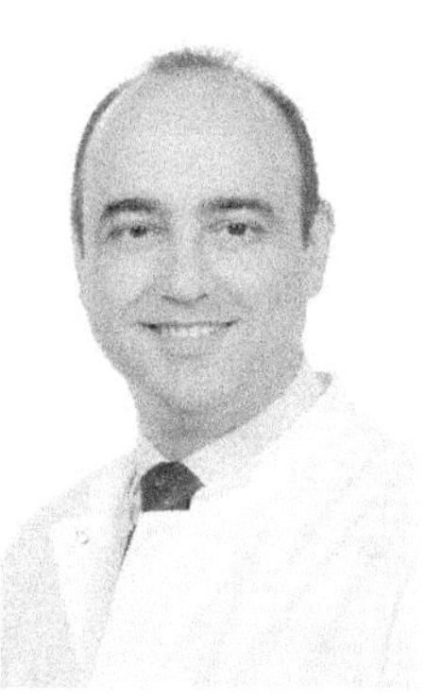 interventional treatment of DVT, PCS, PTS and other vascular diseases. To date, he has authored or co-authored more than 60 scientific publications, abstracts and book chapters. He has given over 100 invited lectures at national and international meetings and is a consultant to many medical device manufacturers.